HYPOTHYROIDISM

DIET COOKBOOK

Delicious And Nutritious Recipes For Boosting Metabolism, And Enhancing Energy Levels

DR ELIAN GRIFFIN

DISCLAIMER

The nutritional recommendations and recipes in this book are meant solely for informative reasons. They are not meant to replace the counsel, diagnosis, or care of a qualified medical expert. If you have any doubts about a medical condition or dietary requirements, you should always see your physician or another trained healthcare expert.

All reasonable efforts have been taken by the author and publisher to ensure that the information contained in this book is correct as of the date of publication. Recommendations may alter, though, as medical knowledge is always changing. When using any of the recipes or instructions found here, the user assumes all liability and assumes no risk, whether personal or otherwise. People who have certain dietary requirements or medical issues should speak with a healthcare provider for personalized guidance. The given recipes are only ideas; you may need to adjust them to suit your own nutritional needs, tastes, and tolerances.

When you use this book, you agree to release the publisher, the author, and their representatives from any liability for any claims, damages, liabilities, costs, or expenditures resulting from your use of the book.

TABLE OF CONTENTS

ABOUT THE BOOK

The "Hypothyroidism Diet Cookbook" is an essential tool for anyone navigating the challenges of managing hypothyroidism through diet. It's important to comprehend how nutrition and thyroid health interact because diet is a major factor in controlling symptoms and promoting general well-being.

This cookbook seeks to arm readers with comprehensive information by first examining hypothyroidism—its causes, symptoms, diagnosis, and available treatments. Next, it explores how diet affects thyroid function, emphasizing the significance of maintaining a healthy, balanced diet.

The foundation of this resource, which describes the nutrients that are necessary for thyroid health and informs readers about foods to eat and avoid. It emphasizes the importance of maintaining a balance between macronutrients (proteins, carbs, and fats) and emphasizes the role that proper hydration and dietary supplements play in promoting thyroid function.

The section on meal planning strategies offers readers sample meal plans that can be customized to accommodate a range of dietary preferences and practical advice on creating menus that support thyroid health. It also includes tips for grocery shopping and meal preparation that are quick and easy to implement, as well as information on how to modify recipes to fit specific needs.

The cookbook's centerpiece, offers a wide range of recipes that have been carefully crafted to improve thyroid health. From nutritious dinners and satisfying snacks to energizing breakfast options, every recipe is formulated to be in line with dietary recommendations for effectively managing hypothyroidism. The recipes also include tips for healthy cooking, ingredient substitutions, and ideas for cooking for family members and friends who have similar health needs.

Beyond diet, lifestyle changes covered highlight holistic approaches to thyroid health. In-depth discussions of subjects like exercise, stress reduction, good sleep hygiene, and mindfulness are included, emphasizing their critical roles in promoting general well-being in addition to dietary changes.

Another major topic covered is weight management, with strategies for healthy weight management specific to hypothyroidism patients. A balanced approach to wellness is emphasized by the helpful advice on goal-setting, progress tracking, and celebrating health milestones that go beyond weight scales.

The book address navigating social situations, eating out, and frequent problems associated with hypothyroidism. These sections offer readers helpful advice on how to maintain dietary discipline while enjoying social contacts and managing particular symptoms like exhaustion and mood swings.

It highlights the significance of long-term management and advocacy for one's health journey. By promoting routine medical exams, continuing education, and creating a community of support, the book equips readers to confidently navigate their thyroid health and proactively adjust their diet as necessary.

The "Hypothyroidism Diet Cookbook" is essentially more than just a cookbook; it's a comprehensive manual that teaches, encourages, and gives people the tools they need to take control of their health through well-informed dietary decisions and holistic lifestyle modifications. This cookbook blends scientific nutrition with practical guidance and personal empowerment to create a useful tool for anyone trying to manage hypothyroidism and maximize their well-being.

CHAPTER ONE

KNOWING ABOUT DIET AND HYPOTHYROIDISM

To manage hypothyroidism, one must understand how specific foods can support thyroid function and reduce symptoms. The thyroid needs certain nutrients, such as iodine, selenium, and zinc, to function optimally.

This cookbook aims to provide recipes rich in these nutrients, helping people with hypothyroidism maintain better health through their diet. Hypothyroidism is a condition where the thyroid gland does not produce enough thyroid hormones, which affects metabolism and overall health.

Understanding the relationship between diet and thyroid function allows people to make informed decisions that support their overall well-being. When it comes to managing hypothyroidism through diet, it's important to stay away from foods that can interfere with thyroid function, like soy products and cruciferous vegetables like broccoli and cabbage. Instead, concentrate on incorporating foods that support thyroid health, like lean proteins, whole grains, and foods rich in vitamins and minerals.

THE ROLE OF DIET IN TREATING HYPOTHYROIDISM

A balanced diet with sufficient amounts of essential nutrients supports thyroid function and can help reduce symptoms like fatigue and weight gain. Nutrition is crucial in managing hypothyroidism, as diet has a direct impact on thyroid hormone production and metabolism.

This cookbook highlights nutrient-dense foods that are good for thyroid health, like seafood for iodine and nuts for selenium.

With a focus on nutrition, people with hypothyroidism can increase their energy levels, better control their weight, and support overall health. This cookbook teaches readers about the significance of selecting foods that support the thyroid gland and how to make thoughtful food choices and maintain a balanced diet to improve overall health and quality of life.

HOW YOU CAN USE THIS COOKBOOK TO HELP

With a variety of recipes that are simple to follow and specifically crafted to support thyroid health, this cookbook for the hypothyroidism diet makes meal planning and preparation easier for those who manage the condition.

Each recipe is carefully selected to include ingredients that are beneficial for thyroid function, ensuring that people can enjoy delicious meals without compromising their dietary needs.

A person can take charge of their diet in a way that supports their thyroid health and general well-being by using this cookbook, which also includes nutritional information for each recipe to help readers make informed decisions about what they eat. Whether you're looking for breakfast ideas, hearty mains, or healthy snacks, this cookbook offers a variety of options that cater to different tastes and dietary preferences.

MAKING EFFECTIVE USE OF THE RECIPES

Planning and selecting recipes that fit your dietary objectives are key to making the most of this cookbook on the hypothyroidism diet. Look through the recipe categories and choose dishes that include thyroid-supportive ingredients such as lean proteins, whole grains, and vitamin- and mineral-rich vegetables.

Pay close attention to the recipes to make sure you're getting the proper ratio of nutrients required for thyroid function.

You can maintain a healthy diet that supports thyroid function and promotes overall wellness by incorporating these recipes into your daily meal planning. Try different recipes to keep meals exciting and enjoyable while still supporting your health goals. All of the recipes in this cookbook are easy to follow and understand.

ADVICE FOR USING THE HYPOTHYROIDISM DIET COOKBOOK SUCCESSFULLY

Use this cookbook as a tool to experiment with new ingredients and cooking methods that support thyroid health.

To succeed with the hypothyroidism diet, you must be consistent and mindful in your food choices. Begin by becoming familiar with the nutritional guidelines provided for each recipe and adjust your meal planning to include a variety of nutrient-dense foods.

Additionally, it's helpful to speak with a doctor or nutritionist to customize your diet plan to your unique requirements and tastes.

Be organized by planning your meals ahead of time and stocking up on ingredients that are necessary for thyroid support. Finally, pay attention to how your body responds to various foods and make necessary dietary adjustments to maximize your health outcomes.

With commitment and the right tools, you can successfully manage hypothyroidism through wholesome and delectable meals made with this cookbook.

CHAPTER TWO

FUNDAMENTALS OF HYPOTHYROIDISM

OVERVIEW OF HYPOTHYROIDISM

Hypothyroidism is a disorder in which the thyroid gland fails to produce enough thyroid hormones to meet the body's needs. Thyroid hormones are essential for controlling energy levels, metabolism, and a host of other bodily functions. Low thyroid hormone levels can cause symptoms like weight gain, dry skin, fatigue, and cold sensitivity. The first step in understanding hypothyroidism is realizing how it affects your overall health and well-being. To start, you should understand that thyroid hormones affect almost every organ system in the body, from heart rate to digestion.

Hypothyroidism management necessitates a multifaceted strategy that frequently involves hormone replacement therapy to replenish the missing hormones. Hormone replacement therapy attempts to return hormone levels to normal, thereby reducing symptoms and averting complications. Dietary adjustments and consistent exercise are also important components of an effective lifestyle; by concentrating on these fundamentals, people can better manage the challenges of living with hypothyroidism and sustain optimal health.

REASONS AND SIGNS

Understanding the causes of hypothyroidism can help patients and healthcare professionals identify the underlying cause of the condition and determine the most appropriate treatment plan. There are many different causes of hypothyroidism, including autoimmune diseases like Hashimoto's thyroiditis, thyroid surgery, radiation therapy, and certain medications. The symptoms of hypothyroidism can vary widely but often include fatigue, weight gain, constipation, dry skin, hair loss, and sensitivity to cold.

Treatment for hypothyroidism usually consists of daily thyroid hormone replacement medication, such as levothyroxine, to restore hormone levels to normal.

Regular monitoring and dosage adjustments may be required to ensure optimal thyroid function and symptom management. Diagnosing hypothyroidism involves a combination of medical history, physical examination, and laboratory tests. Blood tests that measure thyroid hormone levels, particularly TSH (thyroid-stimulating hormone) and T4 (thyroxine), are essential for confirming a diagnosis.

OPTIONS FOR DIAGNOSIS AND TREATMENT

When diagnosing hypothyroidism, a patient's medical history is a vital tool in determining risk factors and underlying causes. Symptoms like fatigue, weight gain, dry skin, and cold sensitivity prompt doctors to order specific tests to confirm the diagnosis and rule out other possible conditions. Laboratory tests are also used to measure thyroid hormone levels accurately.

The mainstay of treatment for hypothyroidism is hormone replacement therapy, which involves the use of synthetic thyroid hormones like levothyroxine to supplement the hormones that the thyroid gland is not producing in sufficient amounts. This helps to restore normal metabolic function and effectively manage symptoms. The dosage of thyroid hormone replacement medication is customized to the patient's needs based on the results of blood tests and ongoing symptom assessment. Follow-up appointments and periodic blood tests are required to monitor thyroid hormone levels and make necessary medication dosage adjustments.

DIETARY INFLUENCE ON THYROID FUNCTION

The role of diet in maintaining thyroid health is important, especially for those who have hypothyroidism. Nutrients like iodine, zinc, and selenium are necessary for the production and metabolism of thyroid hormones.

Eating foods high in these nutrients, like seafood, nuts, seeds, and dairy products, can support optimal thyroid function. Another way to support thyroid health is to limit your intake of goitrogens, which are compounds found in some vegetables like kale and cabbage.

A well-balanced diet for hypothyroidism should consist of a range of nutrient-dense foods to guarantee that the body is getting enough vitamins, minerals, and antioxidants. Whole grains, lean proteins, fruits, and vegetables are good sources of nutrients and also contribute to overall health and well-being. It's also important to stay properly hydrated by drinking enough water each day. By emphasizing foods that are high in nutrients and keeping a well-balanced diet, people can support thyroid function and better manage the symptoms of hypothyroidism.

A WELL-BALANCED DIET IS CRUCIAL FOR TREATING HYPOTHYROIDISM

To support thyroid function, metabolism, and energy production—all of which help to alleviate symptoms and improve quality of life—people with hypothyroidism must maintain a balanced diet. This involves a variety of foods that provide essential nutrients, such as vitamins, minerals, protein, and healthy fats.

Nutrient-dense foods, such as lean proteins, whole grains, fruits, and vegetables, ensure adequate intake of essential nutrients while promoting overall health.

Maintaining proper hydration by drinking enough water throughout the day supports optimal metabolic function and overall health. Reducing excessive consumption of refined sugars and processed foods can help stabilize blood sugar levels and prevent fluctuations in energy levels. Balancing macronutrients, including carbohydrates, proteins, and fats, help regulate energy levels and metabolism, which can be disrupted in individuals with hypothyroidism.

A personalized nutrition plan that addresses specific dietary requirements and supports thyroid health can be developed by working with a healthcare provider or registered dietitian. Individuals can optimize thyroid function and enhance overall well-being by focusing on nutrient-rich foods, maintaining a balanced diet, and making healthy lifestyle choices.

CHAPTER THREE

ESSENTIAL DIETARY PRACTICES FOR HYPOTHYROIDISM

ESSENTIAL MINERALS FOR A HEALTHY THYROID

Consuming essential nutrients that support thyroid function is the key to optimal thyroid health. Among these, iodine is particularly important as it is a building block for thyroid hormones; sources include iodized salt, seaweed, and seafood. Selenium is another essential mineral that functions as an antioxidant to help convert thyroid hormones for proper metabolism; good sources include Brazil nuts, fish, and eggs. Zinc is also important for thyroid hormone production and can be found in meat, shellfish, and seeds.

Other necessary vitamins include vitamin D (found in sunshine and fortified foods), B vitamins (particularly B12), iron (found in lean meats, beans, and spinach), and calcium (found in dairy products, meat, and fortified cereals).

Maintaining a healthy balance between these nutrients will help your thyroid function at its best and support your overall health and vitality.

FOODS TO TAKE AND LEAVE OUT

A thyroid-supporting diet emphasizes nourishing foods over inhibiting ones. To support thyroid hormone production, include iodine-rich foods like iodized salt, seafood, and seaweed. Selenium-rich foods like Brazil nuts, fish, and eggs aid in hormone conversion and should be a regular part of your diet. Zinc sources like meat, shellfish, and seeds also play a critical role in thyroid health.

Conversely, minimize foods that can disrupt thyroid function: goitrogens found in cruciferous vegetables (broccoli, cauliflower, cabbage) can inhibit the absorption of iodine if ingested in excess; fermented soy products can also disrupt the production of thyroid hormones; and processed foods high in unhealthy fats and refined sugars should be avoided as they can cause inflammation and eventually disrupt thyroid function.

MACRONUTRIENT (PROTEINS, CARBS, AND FATS) EQUILIBRIUM

Maintaining thyroid health requires a balanced intake of macronutrients, which include proteins, carbohydrates, and fats. Lean meats, fish, legumes, and dairy products are good sources of proteins, while complex carbohydrates, such as those found in whole grains, fruits, and vegetables, provide energy and vital nutrients. Refined sugars should be avoided in excess as they can upset hormone balance and aggravate inflammation.

Hydration is equally important as water supports nutrient transport, waste removal, and overall cellular function. Aim for adequate hydration by drinking water throughout the day and consuming hydrating foods like fruits and vegetables.

Healthy fats, like those found in avocados, nuts, seeds, and olive oil, are crucial for hormone production and overall cellular health.

By balancing these macronutrients, you can contribute to optimal thyroid function and ensure stable energy levels.

THE VALUE OF HYDRATION

Dehydration can impair hormone production and hinder metabolic rate, leading to fatigue and other symptoms. Hydration is crucial for maintaining thyroid function and general health. Water is necessary for controlling body temperature, facilitating nutrient transport, and supporting metabolic processes, all of which have an impact on thyroid function.

Drink eight glasses of water a day or more, depending on your activity level, the weather, and your personal needs. Fruits and vegetables (cucumber, celery, and watermelon) are good sources of water; herbal teas and broths can also help you stay hydrated while supplying extra nutrients. When you stay well hydrated, you can support thyroid health and improve your overall well-being.

Apart from maintaining a well-balanced diet, thyroid function can also be supported by specific dietary supplements. If your diet does not contain enough iodine-rich foods, you can benefit from taking iodine supplements; however, excessive intake of iodine can cause thyroid function to be disrupted.

If your diet does not contain enough selenium-rich foods, such as Brazil nuts or fish, you can benefit from taking selenium supplements. To ensure safety and efficacy, you should speak with a healthcare provider before beginning any supplement regimen.

Omega-3 fatty acids, found in fish oil supplements, can reduce inflammation and support thyroid health; vitamin D supplements are advised if you have insufficient sun exposure or dietary intake; herbal supplements, such as ashwagandha and ginseng, are popular for supporting the thyroid, but their efficacy varies, so see a healthcare professional before use; and

B-complex vitamins, especially B12, support thyroid hormone synthesis.

You can successfully support thyroid function and overall health by using these dietary supplements in conjunction with a balanced diet; periodic thyroid function testing by blood tests is recommended to make necessary adjustments to your regimen and guarantee optimal thyroid health.

CHAPTER FOUR

MEAL PLANNING AND STRATEGIES

HOW TO ARRANGE FOOD FOR OPTIMAL THYROID FUNCTION

Choosing foods that are high in iodine, zinc, and selenium—found in seafood, Brazil nuts, and lean meats—is a good place to start when meal planning for thyroid health. You should also include foods high in vitamin D—found in fortified dairy products or sunshine—because low levels of this nutrient have been linked to thyroid disorders. Finally, foods high in fiber—found in whole grains, fruits, and vegetables— help regulate digestion and metabolism, which in turn supports thyroid health overall.

For optimal planning, think about having small, frequent meals to help stabilize blood sugar and prevent energy dips. Steer clear of goitrogenic foods (such as cabbage, broccoli, and soy products) as these can interfere with thyroid function if consumed in large amounts raw; instead, lightly cook or steam these foods. Finally, drink lots of water and herbal teas to stay hydrated, as dehydration can worsen thyroid symptoms. Finally, by emphasizing nutrient-dense, balanced meals, you can support your thyroid and general health.

MAKING NUTRITIOUS AND BALANCED MENUS

For a hypothyroidism diet, a variety of nutrient-rich foods should be included in menus that are balanced and free of potential triggers. Lean proteins, like those found in poultry, fish, and tofu, are a good place to start because they provide the essential amino acids needed for thyroid function. Complex carbohydrates, like those found in whole grains, sweet potatoes, or quinoa, can be paired with proteins to provide energy throughout the day. Nuts, avocado, and olive oil are good sources of healthy fats that aid in hormone production and the absorption of fat-soluble vitamins.

Aim for a rainbow of nutrients by including as many different colors of fruits and vegetables as possible in each meal.

Leafy greens, such as spinach and kale, are high in vitamins A and C, which support the immune system and thyroid health. You can support thyroid hormone synthesis by including sources of iodine and selenium, such as seaweed, eggs, and Brazil nuts.

You can use herbs and spices, such as turmeric, ginger, and cinnamon, not only for flavor but also for their anti-inflammatory properties, which can help thyroid function.

EXAMPLE DINNER SCHEDULES FOR VARIOUS DIETARY NEEDS

Meal planning can be made easier for people with hypothyroidism by using sample meal plans that cater to various dietary preferences. If you are vegetarian or vegan, try including plant-based proteins like legumes, tofu, and tempeh in your meals. For breakfast, have a smoothie made with almond milk, spinach, berries, and a scoop of plant-based protein powder. For lunch, have a quinoa salad with roasted vegetables, chickpeas, and tahini dressing. For dinner, try a lentil curry with brown rice and steamed broccoli.

If you follow a Mediterranean diet, focus on lean proteins such as grilled chicken or fish served with a range of fresh vegetables and whole grains. Start your day with a Greek yogurt parfait with nuts and honey on top for breakfast; have a Greek salad for lunch that has grilled chicken, mixed greens, feta cheese, and olives; for dinner, try a Mediterranean-style stuffed bell pepper that is topped with ground turkey, quinoa, and herbs and served with roasted vegetables.

ADVICE FOR MEAL PLANNING AND GROCERY SHOPPING

Creating a detailed grocery list based on your meal plan will help you shop more efficiently and avoid making impulsive purchases. Fresh produce, lean proteins, whole grains, and healthy fats should be prioritized over processed foods high in sugar and trans fats. When choosing produce, such as berries and leafy greens, go for organic options to minimize exposure to pesticides that may interfere with thyroid function.

During meal prep, cook large quantities of staples like quinoa, brown rice, and grilled chicken to have on hand for quick, wholesome meals. To keep prepared meals and ingredients fresh and reduce exposure to harmful chemicals found in plastic containers, portion out snacks like sliced vegetables with hummus or yogurt with nuts and berries. Label and date items in the refrigerator and freezer for easy identification and rotation.

RECIPE MODIFICATIONS FOR YOUR NEEDS

Simple substitutions and adjustments can be made to recipes to meet your dietary needs for thyroid health. For example, replace regular salt in soups and salads with iodized salt or sea vegetables like seaweed flakes. To increase fiber and nutrient content, replace refined grains with whole grains like brown rice, quinoa, or oats. Choose recipes that use ingredients rich in iodine, selenium, and vitamin D to support thyroid function.

Use healthy fats like olive oil or avocado oil instead of butter or margarine for cooking and baking; swap out red meats, which can have higher saturated fat content, for lean proteins like chicken breast, turkey, or fish; add lots of leafy greens and vibrant vegetables to meals for extra vitamins and minerals; and experiment with herbs and spices to add flavor without using too much salt or sugar.

RECIPES FOR THYROID HEALTH IN THE MORNING

Start your day off right with these tasty and nutritious thyroid-healthy breakfast options. A substantial meal is important for maintaining energy levels during the day, particularly for people who are managing hypothyroidism. Try including foods high in iodine, selenium, and essential vitamins. A straightforward but powerful breakfast option is a smoothie bowl filled with spinach, berries, Greek yogurt, and chia seeds. This blend offers probiotics, antioxidants, and fiber, which support gut health and thyroid function.

A balanced breakfast that not only fuels your morning but also helps regulate metabolism and hormone production—both crucial for managing the symptoms of hypothyroidism—is a veggie omelet made with eggs, spinach, tomatoes, and a sprinkle of cheese. Eggs are rich in selenium and iodine, and spinach adds a dose of magnesium and fiber.

Pair it with a slice of whole-grain toast topped with avocado for healthy fats and additional fiber.

If you have a sweet tooth, try oatmeal with nuts and seeds and a drizzle of maple syrup or honey. Oats are high in fiber, which helps with digestion and blood sugar regulation. Nuts and seeds add healthy fats and proteins to the oatmeal, making it a filling and thyroid-supporting breakfast that keeps you going until lunch.

LUNCH IDEAS TO INCREASE VITALITY

Lunch is a chance to replenish energy and refuel, which is particularly crucial for hypothyroidism sufferers. Choose nutrient-dense meals that give you sustained energy without spiking your blood sugar.

For example, a salad full of leafy greens, grilled chicken or salmon, quinoa, and a rainbow of vibrant vegetables is a great option. Leafy greens are full of vitamins and minerals, including iron and vitamin C, which are critical for thyroid function.

A whole-grain wrap stuffed with lean protein (like turkey or tofu), mixed greens, avocado, and hummus is another filling option. Whole grains offer complex carbohydrates that release energy gradually, keeping you full and focused all afternoon. The avocado adds healthy fats and potassium, and the hummus supplies fiber and plant-based protein that supports gut health.

Vegetable and lentil soup is a warm, comforting lunch option. Rich in fiber and protein, lentils aid in digestion and release energy gradually. Serve with whole-grain bread or crackers for extra fiber and complex carbohydrates. This filling soup not only satisfies hunger but also supports thyroid function by providing necessary nutrients and stable energy levels.

RICH IN NUTRIENT DINNERS TO SUPPORT THE THYROID

A balanced dinner option would be a grilled salmon fillet served with roasted sweet potatoes and steamed broccoli. Salmon is rich in omega-3 fatty acids, which have anti-inflammatory properties and support thyroid hormone production. Sweet potatoes are full of fiber and vitamin A, while broccoli provides antioxidants and essential nutrients like vitamin C. Dinner is an opportunity to enjoy flavorful meals that support thyroid health and overall well-being. Focus on nutrient-dense ingredients that provide essential vitamins and minerals.

Stir-fried tofu or chicken with quinoa and colorful veggies like bell peppers, carrots, and snap peas make a delicious dinner idea as well. Lean protein is provided by the tofu and chicken, while quinoa provides complete proteins and complex carbohydrates. The vegetables add fiber, vitamins, and minerals, and the meal is well-rounded to support thyroid function and general health.

Serve a turkey or lentil chili with brown rice or whole-grain bread for a hearty and filling supper. Both turkey and lentils are great sources of lean protein and fiber, which helps with digestion and gives you long-lasting energy.

The chili's tomatoes and beans are packed with vital nutrients and antioxidants that help with thyroid function and overall wellness.

SMOOTHIES AND SNACKS FOR A BALANCED DIET

Snacking is a great way to increase energy and sate cravings in between meals, which is particularly beneficial for people with hypothyroidism. Choose high-nutrient snacks that offer a mix of fiber, healthy fats, and protein. A handful of mixed nuts and seeds is a quick and filling snack; walnuts and almonds are particularly high in selenium and omega-3 fatty acids, which support thyroid function and lower inflammation.

Another delicious snack idea is Greek yogurt topped with fresh berries and a sprinkle of granola. Greek yogurt is high in protein and probiotics, which support immune function and gut health. Berries are full of vitamins and antioxidants, and the granola adds crunch and extra fiber. This snack not only satisfies hunger but also provides vital nutrients for thyroid health.

A green smoothie made with spinach, kale, banana, and almond milk is a tasty way to increase nutrient intake and support thyroid health throughout the day. Leafy greens like spinach and kale are rich in vitamins A and K, which are essential for thyroid function and overall health. A banana adds natural sweetness and potassium, and almond milk adds creaminess without dairy.

SWEETS AND SNACKS THAT ARE SAFE FOR YOUR THYROID

Decadent yet healthful dessert options include dark chocolate avocado mousse, which combines the benefits of dark chocolate (which offers antioxidants and mood-boosting properties) and avocado (which provides healthy fats and potassium) with a hint of honey or maple syrup for sweetness.

Eating desserts and treats can still be part of a thyroid-friendly diet as long as they are consumed in moderation and with nutrient-dense foods and minimal refined sugar intake.

Another guilt-free dessert option is coconut milk-based chia seed pudding with fresh fruit on top. Rich in fiber and omega-3 fatty acids, chia seeds support stable blood sugar levels and digestive health; coconut milk adds creaminess and healthy fats; fresh fruit offers natural sweetness and vital vitamins; this dessert not only satisfies sweet tooths but also supplies nutrients that are good for thyroid health.

A tasty and thyroid-friendly dessert that cools you down on hot days while providing essential nutrients is homemade fruit sorbet made with frozen berries and a dash of citrus juice. Berries are rich in vitamins and antioxidants, and citrus fruits like lemons and limes add brightness and flavor without added sugars. Blend until smooth.

CHAPTER FIVE

COOKING METHODS AND ADVICE

RECIPES FOR HEALTHIER COOKING FOR THE THYROID

It's important to prioritize cooking techniques that maintain nutrients while minimizing the need for added fats and sugars. For example, steaming vegetables is a great way to retain their vitamins and minerals without using extra oils or seasonings. You can also bake, grill, or sauté food with a small amount of coconut oil or olive oil, which both provide healthy fats that are beneficial for thyroid function. Slow cooking is another great technique that keeps food moist and full of nutrients while allowing flavors to blend harmoniously.

Including whole foods such as lean proteins, whole grains, and a rainbow of colorful vegetables is essential. Steaming fish, for example, retains its delicate flavors and its omega-3 fatty acids; you can flavor it further with fresh herbs and a squeeze of lemon juice. Roasting vegetables can also enhance their natural sweetness and make them more appetizing, especially for those who may find them boring. Turmeric, garlic, and ginger are examples of herbs and spices that not only add flavor but also have anti-inflammatory properties that support thyroid health.

High-heat cooking methods, such as deep-frying, should be avoided because they can degrade nutrients and produce unhealthy compounds. Instead, use low-heat methods, like poaching, to keep food moist and tender without using extra fat. Pressure cooking is also a great option, as it can save a lot of cooking time without sacrificing nutrients. Finally, when cooking grains and legumes, think about using techniques like soaking and sprouting to improve digestibility and nutrient absorption, making your meals easy to digest and full of nutrients.

EXCHANGES OF INGREDIENTS AND SUBSTITUTIONS

Making wise substitutions when cooking for hypothyroidism can improve the nutritional value of your meals without compromising on flavor.

For example, you can increase the amount of fiber in your dishes by using whole grain flours like almond flour, coconut flour, or whole wheat flour; you can lower cholesterol and add omega-3 fatty acids by using flaxseed meal or chia seeds in place of eggs in baking. These substitutions also preserve the desired texture and flavor of your food.

In place of dairy, try lower-saturated-fat alternatives like almond milk, coconut yogurt, or cashew cheese; if you like creamy sauces, pureeing soaked cashews or avocados to produce a rich, creamy texture without dairy; use natural sweeteners like honey, maple syrup, or stevia to cut back on refined sugar intake while enhancing flavor in your recipes; and swapping out white rice for quinoa or brown rice to boost protein and give you a steady release of energy that helps keep your blood sugar levels in check.

Herbs and spices also work well as substitutions. For example, fresh herbs like basil, cilantro, and parsley can boost flavor without adding sodium; spices like cumin, turmeric, and cinnamon not only give a rich flavor to food but also have anti-inflammatory properties that support thyroid function; and using seaweed or kelp instead of regular salt can supply iodine, which is essential for thyroid health. These easy substitutions can make your cooking taste good and support thyroid health.

ENHANCERS OF FLAVOR WITHOUT ENDANGERING HEALTH

The use of natural ingredients and flavor-enhancing cooking methods can enhance flavor without sacrificing health. For example, fresh herbs such as rosemary, thyme, and oregano can improve the flavor profile of your food without adding excessive salt or artificial seasonings. Citrus zest, like lemon, lime, or orange, adds a burst of freshness that brightens any dish, from salads to grilled meats. Garlic and onion, which not only enhance flavor but also have immune-boosting properties, can be used to add savory depth to your food.

Another great way to add flavor is to add spices. For example, turmeric, which adds color and health benefits, can be added to soups, curries, stews, and smoothies. Cumin and coriander, on the other hand, give stews and curries a warm, earthy flavor. Paprika gives roasted vegetables a smoky depth. Finally, adding seaweed, such as kelp or nori, can naturally add umami flavor to soups and stir-fries, thereby reducing the need for MSG or other artificial flavor enhancers.

The use of natural sweeteners like honey, agave nectar, or maple syrup can add a subtle sweetness to dishes, balancing flavors without the refined sugars found in processed foods. These strategies allow you to enjoy rich, satisfying flavors while keeping your meals thyroid-friendly and health-conscious. Additionally, experimenting with fermented foods can introduce complex flavors and beneficial probiotics to your diet.

COOKING FOR FRIENDS AND FAMILY WHEN YOU'RE HYPOTHYROID

A balanced meal that is both tasty and beneficial for thyroid function can be made by preparing dishes like baked salmon with a side of steamed broccoli and quinoa. If you have family or friends who suffer from hypothyroidism, it's important to create dishes that are both delicious and supportive of their health needs. To start, understand their dietary restrictions and preferences and make sure that each meal is not only nutritious but also enjoyable. Focus on including a variety of foods that support thyroid health, such as iodine-rich seafood, selenium-packed nuts, and antioxidant-rich vegetables.

Easy ways to incorporate thyroid-friendly ingredients into regular meals are to cook with coconut oil or olive oil (better fat choices that promote thyroid health); add flavor with garlic, ginger, and turmeric (which have anti-inflammatory and depth of flavor); add foods like spinach, seaweed, and sweet potatoes (which are high in iodine and other essential nutrients) to salads and sides; and cook with vibrant, colorful food to ensure a good balance of vitamins and minerals.

A variety of herbs and spices can help make meals exciting without adding extra calories or sodium. Making dishes that are naturally sweetened with fruits or using whole grain alternatives can also make the meals more satisfying. By considering these factors, you can make sure that everyone at the table enjoys delicious, healthful meals that support their thyroid health. Don't forget to adjust portion sizes and cooking methods to suit everyone's needs.

TIME-SELECTION ADVICE FOR THE KITCHEN

Creating a foundation of quick and easy meals can be achieved by batch-cooking quinoa, roasting a variety of vegetables, and grilling some chicken breasts. Using time-saving tips in the kitchen can make cooking for thyroid health both efficient and enjoyable. One such tactic is meal prepping. Set aside a few hours every week to chop vegetables, cook grains, and prepare proteins. This preparation not only saves time during the week but also guarantees that you always have nutritious ingredients ready to go.

Slow cookers: They're great for making hearty soups, stews, and casseroles with little hands-on time, allowing flavors to develop beautifully. Pressure cookers: They're great for quickly cooking beans, lentils, and grains, making them a convenient option for nutritious meals. Food processors: They're great for quickly chopping, slicing, and pureeing ingredients, speeding up the preparation process for everything from salads to smoothies.

To further increase efficiency, organize your pantry so that all of your staple ingredients are within easy reach, labeling containers so you can find them quickly. To help you stay on track with your cooking goals, use meal planning apps or make a weekly menu.

CHAPTER SIX

ADJUSTMENTS TO LIFESTYLE FOR THYROID HEALTH

EXERCISE AND PHYSICAL ACTIVITY'S SIGNIFICANCE

Frequent exercise is critical for maintaining thyroid health, particularly for those who are managing hypothyroidism. Physical activity stimulates thyroid gland function and metabolism, which aids in energy management and weight management. Exercises that are beneficial for thyroid function include brisk walking, cycling, and yoga. It is important to find activities that you enjoy and can stick with, as consistency is key to reaping the benefits of exercise for thyroid health.

Including exercise in daily routines can be made easier by beginning with small goals, like taking short walks or doing gentle stretching sessions. People with hypothyroidism can maintain energy levels without becoming overly exhausted by gradually increasing the intensity and duration of their exercise regimen.

It's also crucial to pay attention to your body and take breaks when necessary, as too much exercise may strain your adrenal glands and exacerbate symptoms. People who incorporate regular physical activity into their lifestyle can support thyroid health while also feeling well and full of life.

TECHNIQUES FOR STRESS MANAGEMENT

A routine that includes daily stress-relieving activities, like journaling or spending time in nature, can significantly impact overall health and well-being. It's important to identify personal stress triggers and implement strategies that effectively relieve tension and promote mental clarity. For people with hypothyroidism, stress management is crucial because stress can negatively affect thyroid function and exacerbate symptoms. Techniques like deep breathing exercises, meditation, and mindfulness can help reduce cortisol levels and promote relaxation.

By prioritizing stress management techniques, individuals with hypothyroidism can optimize their thyroid function and improve their quality of life. Long-term benefits of integrating these practices into daily life include improved sleep quality and an overall sense of well-being. Mindfulness practices enable individuals to cultivate awareness of their thoughts and emotions, fostering a sense of calm and resilience in the face of stress. Daily routines can incorporate techniques like progressive muscle relaxation or guided imagery to promote relaxation and reduce anxiety levels.

THE EFFECTS OF SLEEP HYGIENE ON THYROID FUNCTION

A regular sleep schedule, a calming bedtime routine, and optimizing the sleep environment for comfort and darkness are all important components of good sleep hygiene. Refraining from stimulants like caffeine and electronics before bed can help promote restful sleep and improve thyroid function.

Adequate sleep is essential for hormone regulation and cellular repair, which are critical processes for individuals with hypothyroidism.

Creating a sleep-friendly environment, such as keeping the bedroom cool and dark, can enhance sleep quality and support thyroid health. Prioritizing consistent sleep patterns and promptly addressing sleep disturbances can help individuals with hypothyroidism feel more rested and energized throughout the day. By focusing on improving sleep hygiene, individuals can enhance their overall health and well-being while supporting optimal thyroid function. Establishing a calming bedtime routine, such as reading or taking a warm bath, can help the body signal that it's time to unwind.

GOALS FOR WORK AND HEALTH BALANCED

To effectively manage their time and prioritize self-care and health maintenance, people with hypothyroidism must find a balance between their work commitments and health goals. This can be achieved by balancing responsibilities, which can lower stress levels and improve overall well-being. Time management techniques, such as making schedules and assigning tasks to others when needed, can assist people in finding a balance that supports both professional and personal health goals.

A balance between work and health goals can help individuals with hypothyroidism effectively manage their condition and improve their quality of life. Proactively managing stress and prioritizing self-care can lead to improved productivity and sustained energy levels throughout the day. Establishing boundaries and learning to say no to excessive work demands can help individuals with hypothyroidism maintain energy levels and prevent burnout. Including regular breaks and prioritizing self-care activities, such as exercise or relaxation techniques, can support thyroid health and overall well-being.

INCLUDING MINDFULNESS TECHNIQUES

People with hypothyroidism can benefit greatly from mindfulness practices because they foster self-awareness and reduce stress. Activities like body scanning, deep breathing exercises, and mindfulness meditation can help people develop a sense of presence and calm in their daily lives. Mindfulness is the practice of paying attention to thoughts, feelings, and sensations without passing judgment.

Including meditation or mindfulness exercises in daily routines can be accomplished by scheduling specific times for these activities. Developing a regular practice that supports thyroid health can be facilitated by starting small and working your way up to longer sessions. Mindfulness techniques can also be incorporated into everyday activities, like mindful eating or walking, to increase awareness and promote relaxation. Hypothyroidism sufferers who regularly practice mindfulness can lower their stress levels, increase mental clarity, and support thyroid function overall.

CHAPTER SEVEN

CONTROLLING WEIGHT IN HYPOTHYROID PATIENTS

RECOGNIZING THE DIFFICULTIES OF WEIGHT MANAGEMENT

Because thyroid hormone imbalances have a unique effect on metabolism, managing weight with hypothyroidism can present unique challenges. For example, hypothyroidism frequently results in a slower metabolic rate, which makes weight gain easier and weight loss harder.

Additionally, fluid retention and increased sensitivity to carbohydrates can complicate weight management efforts. Recognizing these challenges is essential to creating effective strategies that are customized to each individual's needs.

Managing stress levels and making sure you get enough sleep can help optimize thyroid function and support weight management efforts.

By addressing these factors comprehensively, people with hypothyroidism can better navigate the difficulties associated with weight management. To address these challenges, focusing on a balanced diet that supports thyroid function is essential. This includes incorporating foods rich in iodine, selenium, and zinc, which are important for thyroid hormone production and metabolism regulation.

TECHNIQUES FOR MAINTAINING OR LOSING WEIGHT HEALTHILY

A thyroid-friendly diet that emphasizes whole grains, lean proteins, fruits, and vegetables while limiting processed foods and refined sugars is a key strategy for healthy weight loss or maintenance with hypothyroidism.

This dietary approach not only supports thyroid function but also promotes overall health and sustainable weight management. In addition, regular physical activity and lifestyle modifications are important.

Another essential element is regular exercise. Although hypothyroidism may make weight loss more difficult, aerobic exercises such as yoga, walking, or swimming can increase metabolism and improve general fitness levels; the key is to begin slowly and increase intensity gradually to prevent overdoing it. Moreover, reducing stress with deep breathing exercises or meditation can support thyroid health and help with weight management efforts.

HAVING REASONABLE OBJECTIVES

Setting realistic goals is essential to managing weight successfully with hypothyroidism. Achievable targets that account for the difficulties caused by thyroid dysfunction should be established.

If weight loss is not the primary goal, then focusing on weight maintenance should be the goal. Non-scale victories like better energy, better sleep, or increased physical fitness should also be taken into consideration when setting realistic goals.

For individualized goal-setting based on metabolic needs and individual health status, it is helpful to speak with a registered dietitian or healthcare professional who specializes in thyroid health. Individuals with hypothyroidism can stay motivated and dedicated to their weight management journey by setting realistic goals and routinely tracking their progress.

TRACKING DEVELOPMENT AND MODIFICATIONS

Effective weight management for people with hypothyroidism requires regular monitoring of progress and making necessary adjustments. Keeping a regular record of food intake, physical activity, and weight fluctuations can give important information about what's working and what may need to be adjusted. This process also helps people see patterns, such as how certain foods or activities affect energy levels or weight fluctuations.

To track progress, it is important to pay attention to changes in mood, sleep quality, and general energy levels in addition to the scale.

Dietary changes, exercise routine modifications, or the exploration of additional stress management strategies are examples of adjustments that may be necessary. People who are proactive and flexible can maximize their efforts at managing their weight despite the difficulties that hypothyroidism presents.

HONORING OFF-SCALE ACHIEVEMENTS

Non-scale victories are achievements that go beyond weight changes, like increased stamina during workouts, better fitting clothes, or improved overall well-being. These achievements are significant indicators of success and should be acknowledged and celebrated throughout the journey. Celebrating non-scale victories is an important part of keeping motivation high and recognizing progress in weight management with hypothyroidism.

Celebrating non-scale victories also helps build confidence and resilience, empowering people to stick to their health goals despite the challenges posed by thyroid dysfunction.

People with hypothyroidism can change their perspective from relying solely on numbers on the scale to appreciating the holistic benefits of their efforts. This approach promotes a positive mindset and reinforces healthy behaviors that support long-term weight management and overall wellness.

CHAPTER EIGHT

SUGGESTIONS FOR DINING OUT WHEN HYPOTHYROID

Managing hypothyroidism can make eating out difficult, but there are ways to enjoy eating out while taking care of your thyroid. To start, look for restaurants that serve healthier options, such as grilled or steamed dishes instead of fried ones. When placing your order, request dressings and sauces on the side to control portions of fats and sugars, which can affect thyroid function. Finally, choose dishes that are high in lean proteins, whole grains, and vegetables to support general health.

Plan: If at all possible, look up the restaurant's menu online. Look for dishes that are lower in sodium because too much salt can interfere with the production of thyroid hormones. Be aware of hidden sources of iodine, like dairy and seafood, as these can affect thyroid function in some people.

When in doubt, ask your server about ingredients or preparation methods to make sure they meet your dietary requirements.

Finally, keep in mind that sugary drinks and too much caffeine can interfere with thyroid function, so stay hydrated with water or herbal teas instead. You can support thyroid health while dining out by being an informed consumer and standing up for your needs.

GETTING AROUND RESTAURANT MENUS

When navigating restaurant menus for hypothyroidism, it's important to be mindful of ingredients and preparation techniques that may affect thyroid function. To start, look for dishes that include lean proteins (such as chicken, turkey, or tofu) and that are baked, steamed, or grilled instead of fried. These healthier cooking methods help to maintain thyroid health.

Eat less seafood and iodized salt, as these high-iodine foods can negatively impact thyroid function; instead, try dishes made with whole grains, such as brown rice or quinoa, which provide fiber and nutrients that are vital for thyroid health in general; vegetables are also a great source of thyroid-supporting antioxidants and vitamins.

You can enjoy dining out while supporting thyroid health by being informed and making thoughtful choices. When reading menu descriptions, keep an eye out for hidden sources of sugar and saturated fats, which can lead to weight gain and metabolic changes associated with hypothyroidism. You can also customize your order by asking for substitutions or modifications to better suit your dietary needs.

ORGANIZING THYROID-FRIENDLY EVENTS

Throwing a thyroid-friendly party means organizing meals that will satisfy hypothyroidism-accompanying guests while providing tasty and nourishing options for all. To begin, try including a range of whole foods on your menu, such as fruits, vegetables, lean proteins, and whole grains; these foods offer vital nutrients, including vitamins, minerals, and antioxidants, that support thyroid function.

To accommodate guests with special dietary needs, think about providing a variety of low-iodine dishes, such as vegetarian or non-seafood options; reduce the amount of added fats and oils in your food by using techniques like grilling, roasting, or steaming; and give guests the option to customize their meals with salad bars and a variety of toppings and dressings on the side.

With careful planning and consideration of your guests' dietary preferences and restrictions, you can host a thyroid-friendly gathering that supports health and well-being for everyone.

When serving beverages, offer hydrating and health-promoting alternatives to alcohol, such as herbal teas, infused water, or fresh juices. Be mindful of ingredients like soy and gluten that can affect thyroid function in some individuals and provide alternatives when possible.

For those who suffer from hypothyroidism, it is important to know how alcohol affects thyroid function. Although moderate alcohol use may not directly impact thyroid hormone production, excessive alcohol use can interfere with medication efficacy and aggravate symptoms like weight gain and fatigue. Alcohol also disturbs sleep patterns, which are critical for hormone regulation and thyroid function in general.

Alcohol's dehydrating effects and potential interactions with thyroid medications should be considered by those managing hypothyroidism. If you choose to drink, stick to lower-alcohol options like wine or light beer, and don't exceed the recommended daily intake of one drink for women and two for men, as per health guidelines.

To stay hydrated and support thyroid health, try these alcohol-free alternatives to cocktails or sparkling water with a splash of fruit juice during social gatherings. If you are concerned about alcohol consumption and its effect on your thyroid medication, speak with your healthcare provider for specific advice.

MANAGING SOCIAL CIRCUMSTANCES CONFIDENTLY

Managing your hypothyroidism while navigating social situations requires you to be an advocate for your health and make educated decisions. To start, let hosts or restaurant personnel know about your dietary preferences and restrictions in advance so they can make accommodations for you. If you're going to a party where there aren't many food options, think about bringing a dish that fits your needs so you can make sure you have something to eat.

Put more emphasis on interacting with people and having fun than just eating and drinking. Take part in discussions or activities that help you relax and de-stress because long-term stress negatively affects thyroid function. Pay attention to your energy levels and give self-care routines like getting enough sleep and exercising regularly priority to support thyroid health in general.

Take breaks as needed and pay attention to your body's signals to maintain balance and well-being throughout social gatherings. If alcohol is served at social events, be mindful of your intake and choose alternatives like herbal teas or sparkling water to stay hydrated and prevent potential interactions with thyroid medications. By standing up for yourself and making thoughtful decisions, you can support the health of your thyroid and navigate social situations with confidence.

CHAPTER NINE

HANDLING LETHARGY AND LOW ENERGY

Among the practical strategies for managing fatigue and low energy levels when managing hypothyroidism are: first, making sure you get enough sleep every night—aim for 7-9 hours of restful sleep to support your body's energy levels and general well-being—as well as developing a relaxing bedtime routine and regular sleep schedule.

Second, eating a well-balanced, nutrient-dense diet is crucial. Pay attention to how lean proteins, whole grains, fruits, and vegetables are included in your meals. Steer clear of refined carbohydrates and sugary foods to help stabilize your energy levels throughout the day. Finally, drinking lots of water to stay hydrated is crucial for sustaining energy and avoiding dehydration, which exacerbates fatigue.

Last but not least, adding regular exercise to your schedule will help you feel more energized and less fatigued. Pick enjoyable and manageable activities like swimming, yoga, or walking. Exercise improves mood, circulation, and sleep quality—all of which are important for effectively managing fatigue.

HANDLING DEPRESSION AND MOOD SWINGS

A multimodal strategy is needed to manage depression and mood swings brought on by hypothyroidism. First and foremost, you must stay in constant contact with your healthcare provider so that they can monitor your hormone levels and make necessary adjustments to your thyroid medication dosage. Good medication management can greatly reduce depressive symptoms and mood swings.

Second, if you include stress-reduction methods into your daily routine, you'll be able to better control your mood swings. Activities and interests that make you happy and fulfilled, as well as stress-reduction techniques like yoga, deep breathing exercises, and mindfulness meditation, can all help you relax and feel better.

Having a strong support system of friends, family, or support groups can also help you feel less alone and more supported emotionally. Speaking candidly with people who share your experiences and feelings can also help you feel less alone and isolated. Getting professional counseling or therapy can also help you develop coping mechanisms and address underlying emotional issues related to hypothyroidism.

TIPS FOR HAIR AND SKIN CARE

Adopting a skincare and haircare regimen that emphasizes hydration and nourishment is essential to maintaining healthy hair and skin when managing hypothyroidism. For skincare, products with hyaluronic acid and ceramides can support skin barrier function and improve moisture retention. Using gentle cleansers and moisturizers appropriate for your skin type can help maintain hydration and prevent dryness.

A weekly deep conditioning treatment or hair mask can help nourish and strengthen your hair. Avoiding excessive heat styling and using heat protectant products when styling can help minimize damage and maintain hair health. Sulfate-free shampoos and conditioners can help prevent dryness and breakage.

Drinking lots of water can help maintain skin elasticity and moisture retention, which is important for hair and skin care. A diet high in vitamins and minerals, like vitamin C, vitamin E, and omega-3 fatty acids, can also support healthy skin and hair. A dermatologist or trichologist can provide customized recommendations based on your individual needs and concerns.

TAKING A TRIP WITH HYPOTHYROID

A copy of your prescription and any pertinent medical records should be packed, as well as an adequate supply of your thyroid medication. Make sure your medication is stored in its original packaging and carry it in your carry-on luggage to prevent loss or damage. Traveling with hypothyroidism requires careful planning to ensure you manage your condition effectively while away from home.

Second, if you're traveling across multiple time zones, take into account the differences in time zones. Speak with your healthcare provider to modify your medication schedule to keep your treatment consistent. You can also set reminders or alarms on your phone to help you remember to take your medication on time.

A medical alert card or bracelet indicating your hypothyroidism should be carried with you or worn in case of emergency. To support your overall health and well-being while traveling, stay hydrated and maintains a balanced diet.

Additionally, research local pharmacies and medical facilities at your destination in case you need to refill your prescription or seek medical assistance.

Managing the interactions between thyroid medication and diet requires awareness of specific foods and supplements that can disrupt thyroid function. To begin with, stay away from consuming large amounts of soy-based products because soy contains compounds called isoflavones that can disrupt the absorption of thyroid hormones. Instead, consume soy products in moderation and at a time other than when you take your thyroid medication.

Second, limit your intake of raw or uncooked cassava, millet, and rutabaga; these foods also contain goitrogens that can interfere with thyroid hormone production. When it comes to cruciferous vegetables, cooking helps reduce the goitrogens that can interfere with thyroid hormone production.

A doctor's advice should always be sought before beginning any new supplement or medication to ensure that it won't conflict with your thyroid treatment. Iron, calcium, and magnesium- or aluminum-containing antacids are among the supplements and medications that can also interfere with the absorption of thyroid medication. Take these supplements at least four hours apart from your thyroid medication to minimize potential interactions.

You can effectively manage your hypothyroidism and support your general health and well-being by being aware of these interactions and making educated decisions about your diet and medication schedule. You should also regularly communicate with your healthcare provider to monitor your thyroid hormone levels and make any necessary adjustments to your treatment plan for the best possible management of your condition.

CHAPTER TEN

SUSTAINING THYROID HEALTH OVER THE LONG TERM

THE VALUE OF ROUTINE MEDICAL EXAMINATIONS

To effectively manage hypothyroidism, medical professionals must schedule regular check-ups to monitor thyroid hormone levels and evaluate overall health. During these visits, blood tests may be performed to measure thyroid-stimulating hormone (TSH), T4, and T3 levels, which provide important insights into thyroid function and allow for necessary dosage adjustments to maintain optimal hormone balance. In addition to monitoring thyroid function, these check-ups also involve monitoring other health indicators, such as blood pressure, cholesterol, and heart function, all of which are frequently impacted by thyroid imbalances. By identifying any abnormalities early on, routine check-ups can prevent potential complications and enable timely intervention.

Diet plays a significant role in managing hypothyroidism, as certain nutrients support thyroid function and overall well-being. As thyroid function changes, adjusting your diet accordingly can help optimize hormone levels and alleviate symptoms. For instance, iodine is crucial for thyroid hormone production, so ensuring adequate intake of iodine-rich foods like seafood, dairy products, and iodized salt is essential. Additionally, incorporating selenium from sources like Brazil nuts, whole grains, and lean meats supports thyroid hormone synthesis and metabolism. Moreover, maintaining a balanced diet rich in fruits, vegetables, and lean proteins provides essential vitamins and minerals that support overall health and immune function. Monitoring dietary changes and their effects on symptoms, such as fatigue or weight gain, helps tailor your diet to better support thyroid health. Consulting with a registered dietitian or healthcare provider can provide personalized guidance on adjusting your diet to complement thyroid treatment and promote overall well-being.

RESEARCH AND ONGOING EDUCATION

Staying informed about hypothyroidism through ongoing education and research empowers individuals to make informed decisions about their health. Advances in medical research continually provide new insights into thyroid disorders, treatment options, and lifestyle management strategies. Keeping up-to-date with credible sources such as medical journals, reputable websites, and healthcare professionals ensures that individuals have access to the latest information and treatment developments. Furthermore, participating in thyroid awareness campaigns and support groups fosters a community where individuals can share experiences, resources, and tips for managing hypothyroidism effectively. Educating oneself about the condition helps individuals advocate for their health needs and collaborate more effectively with healthcare providers.

By staying informed and engaged, individuals can navigate their thyroid health journey with confidence and make proactive decisions that support their overall well-being.

CREATING A NETWORK OF SUPPORT

Creating a network of support is crucial for both emotional and practical assistance during the management of hypothyroidism. Reaching out to friends, family, or support groups that are cognizant of the difficulties associated with having a thyroid condition can offer motivation, empathy, and guidance. Exchanging stories and coping mechanisms for managing symptoms, medication adjustments, and lifestyle modifications promote a sense of community and lessens feelings of isolation. Including loved ones in your medical journey can also help them comprehend the effects of hypothyroidism on day-to-day living and provide invaluable support during trying times. Getting professional counseling or therapy can also offer a secure setting for discussing emotional difficulties and formulating coping mechanisms.

Celebrating milestones and achievements in managing hypothyroidism is important for maintaining motivation and acknowledging personal progress. Whether it's achieving optimal thyroid hormone levels, adopting healthier lifestyle habits, or effectively managing symptoms, recognizing these accomplishments boosts self-esteem and reinforces positive behaviors. Setting small, achievable goals and tracking progress over time provides a sense of accomplishment and encourages continued dedication to thyroid health.

Celebrating successes can take many forms, such as treating yourself to something special, sharing achievements with loved ones, or reflecting on personal growth and resilience. Moreover, taking time to appreciate the improvements in quality of life and overall well-being that come with effective thyroid management reinforces the importance of ongoing self-care and perseverance. By celebrating your health journey, you affirm your commitment to self-improvement and inspire others facing similar challenges to stay proactive and optimistic about their thyroid health.